BECOMING MOTHER

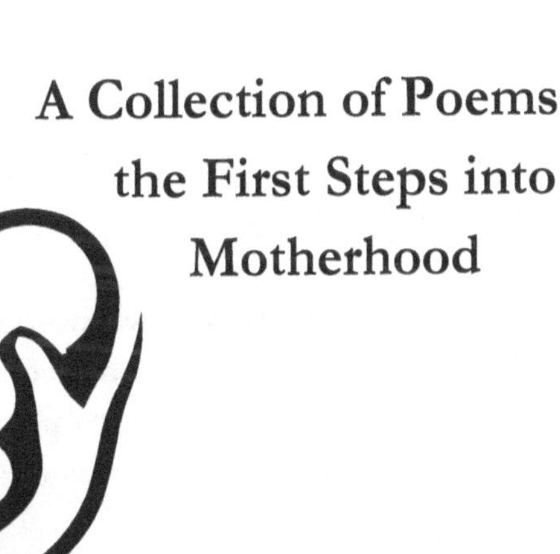

A Collection of Poems on the First Steps into Motherhood

Taylor Quill

Copyright Page
© 2024 by Taylor Quill

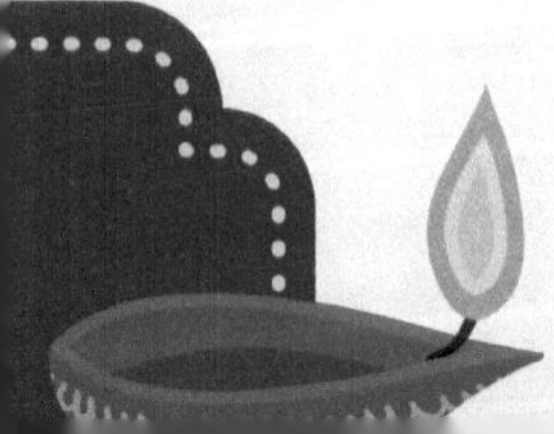

TABLE OF CONTENTS

$\rightarrow$

$\rightarrow$

CHAPTER ONE

"The Whisper of Beginnings"

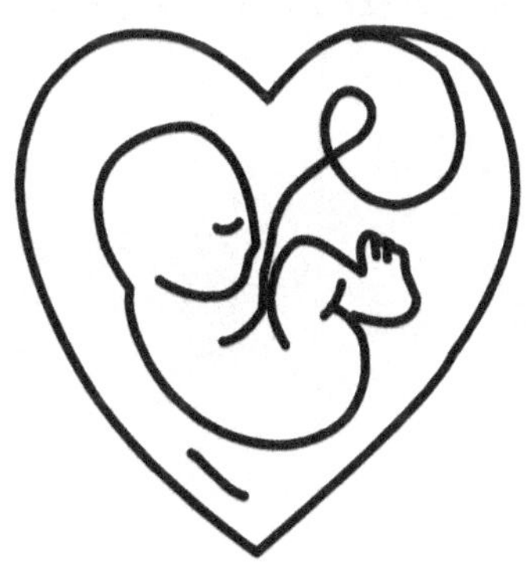

The First Taste of Knowing

A whisper soft, a tender hint,
The taste of life on lips that glint.
A secret shared, a gentle sigh,
As new hope stirs beneath the sky.

Your future swirls in morning light,
A seedling growing through the night.
My heart, it beats a softer tune,
The taste of love, a sweet monsoon.

The world ahead is crisp and clear,
A new life close, forever near.
I see you now, I feel you grow,
The taste of motherhood starts to flow.

The Silent Promise

Beneath the quiet, still and deep,
A promise blooms where shadows sleep.
The softest sound, a rhythmic beat,
The pulse of life that feels so sweet.

I hear the world in whispered tones,
A future shaped in silent stones.
The air is thick with dreams unknown,
Yet still, I taste the seed you've sown.

I see you in the quiet dawn,
A vision bright, a light reborn.
And in my heart, this truth now sings,
A mother's love, the first soft wings.

A Dream Unfolding

I see your face in every dream,
A soft embrace, a perfect gleam.
You're here in silence, far away,
A dream I hold, come what may.

The feel of you is all I know,
A gentle pulse, a steady glow.
I feel you stir, a warmth untold,
A love that's deeper than the cold.

I dream of hands that fit in mine,
A tiny form, a pure design.
A future that I can't yet hold,
But in my heart, your name is bold.

The Softest Touch

The first touch of hope, a glimmer bright,
A dream of you, my heart alight.
Your presence lingers in the air,
A soft caress that's always there.

I feel you, though you're far away,
A quiet voice that starts to sway.
The taste of joy is sweet and true,
It rises high, like morning dew.

I see you in the stars above,
Your life, your light, a gift of love.
I hear your heart inside my soul,
A rhythm that will make me whole.

The First Flicker

I feel the flicker in my soul,
A spark of life that makes me whole.
A warmth that spreads, a rush of light,
Your heartbeat whispers in the night.

I hear your voice, though you're not here,
A sound of love that draws me near.
The taste of change is sweet and wild,
A love that grows inside, a child.

I see you in the morning haze,
A tiny dream that sets the blaze.
The world will shift, but I will stay,
And hold you close, come what may.

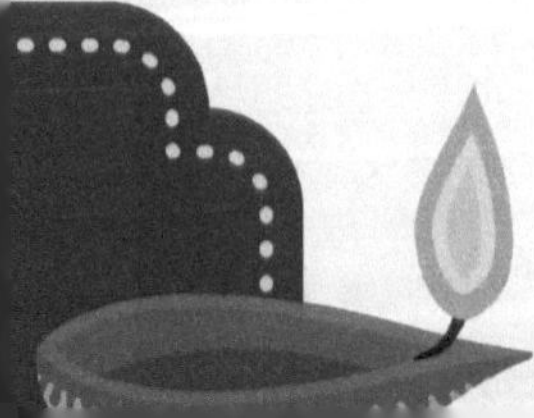

CHAPTER TWO

"Growing Within"

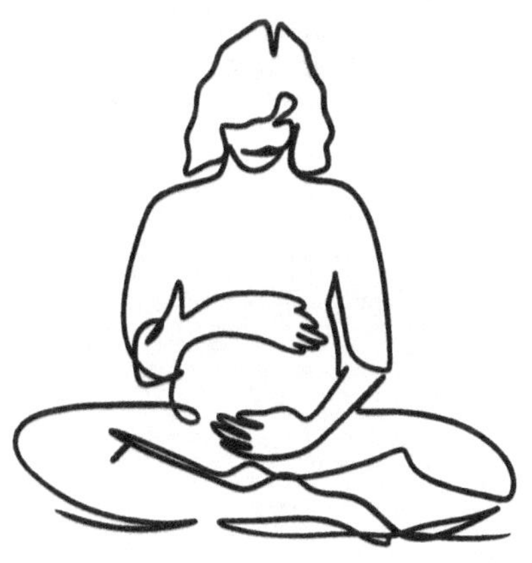

The First Flutter

A flutter soft, a gentle tease,
A breath of wind through autumn trees.
I feel you stir, so light, so pure,
A silent whisper, I'm sure.

Your tiny dance, so sweet, so slight,
A quiet spark in the hush of night.
I hear the promise in your beat,
A rhythm rising, soft and sweet.

I see you, though you're still unseen,
A part of me, a living dream.
The taste of joy begins to grow,
A bond we share, and soon will know.

Beneath My Skin

Beneath my skin, a secret stirs,
A pulse of life, a rhythm blurs.
I feel the change, both soft and strong,
A quiet hum, a lifelong song.

I taste the air, it's richer now,
My body shifts, I don't know how.
But in your flutter, I can tell—
We're two, yet one, in this new shell.

I hear the whispers of your soul,
Your tiny heart that makes me whole.
A love that grows, unseen, untold,
My heart is yours, my hands you'll hold.

The Growing Glow

My body blooms, so soft, so slow,
A tender curve, a gentle glow.
I taste the sweetness of this change,
A world of wonder, wide and strange.

Your presence fills each quiet space,
I feel your dance, I see your face.
The scent of life is all around,
A love that has no end or bound.

I hear your heartbeat, soft and true,
A song that hums in shades of blue.
In every breath, I sense you here,
A bond that holds, so crystal clear.

The Silent Touch

I feel you like a quiet song,
A melody that hums along.
Your tiny whispers stir the air,
A touch I feel, though you're not there.

My body shifts, a gift so bright,
Each change a step in our shared flight.
The taste of life is sharp and sweet,
A new existence we will meet.

I see your presence in the night,
A soft embrace, a gentle light.
In every move, in every breath,
We're bound in love that conquers death.

Growing Together

A curve appears, my body sways,
A quiet shift, in wondrous ways.
I taste the change in every bite,
As life expands within my sight.
I feel you dance, a spark, a leap,

Your tiny steps in rhythm deep.
The world grows wide, so vast, so sweet,
With every pulse, our hearts do meet.

I hear the flutter, soft and light,
A secret song that fills the night.
We grow together, you and I,
Beneath the earth, beneath the sky.

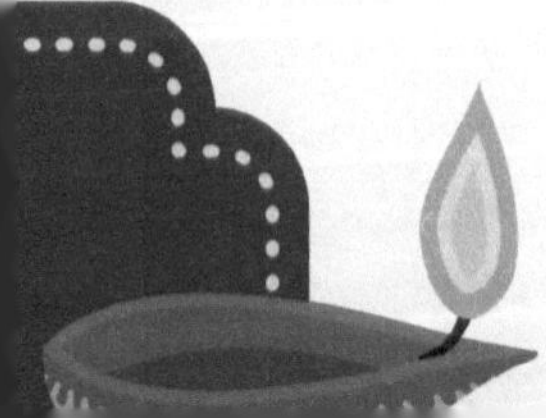

CHAPTER THREE

"A Love Unseen"

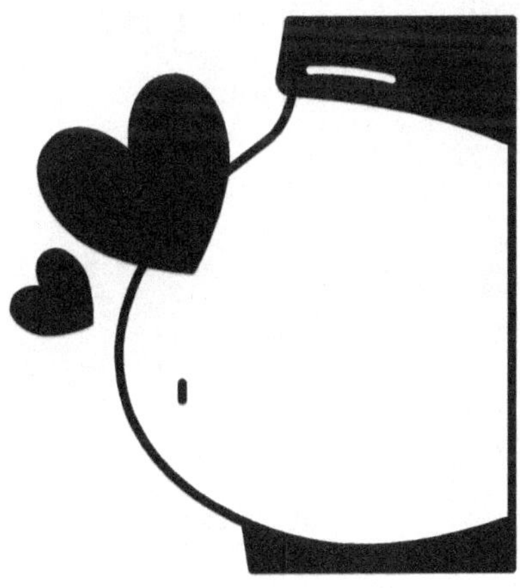

Dreams of You

I wonder what your eyes will be,
Bright as stars or soft as sea.
Will you laugh with joy or cry in fear,
A smile so sweet, so crystal clear?

I see your face in every dream,
A future born of hope's bright gleam.
The taste of love, both soft and strong,
A melody that hums along.

I hear your voice, though you're not here,
A whisper in the wind so near.
Your spirit calls to me each day,
A love I'll never turn away.

The Future You

What will you be, my little one?
A star that rises with the sun?
A gentle heart, a tender soul,
A dreamer who will make us whole?

I taste your name in every breath,
A whisper soft, defying death.
The world awaits with arms outstretched,
A life so full, so tightly etched.

I feel you in my every move,
A bond that can't be stripped or proved.
In your heart, the universe—
A future bright, a loving verse.

Unseen Love

I've never seen your face, my dear,
But love for you is pure, sincere.
I feel you in each gentle beat,
A love so vast, so true, complete.

What will you look like when we meet?
Will you dance, or will you sleep?
I see you in the moonlit sky,
A future bright, too grand to deny.

The taste of love is rich, divine,
A flavor soft, forever mine.
In every breath, I hold you near,
A promise made, a life sincere.

The Heart That Waits

What will you be when you arrive?
A spark of life that makes me thrive?
I feel the pull, the heartstrings play,
A future formed in every day.

I hear you in the silence now,
Your whispers soft, a sacred vow.
I taste the air, it's sweet and true,
A world of love I'll give to you.

I see your future far ahead,
A life of joy, of dreams well-spread.
Though we've yet to meet, my love is real,
A promise formed, a love I feel.

A Love That Knows

Though I've not seen your face or form,
My heart knows you, soft and warm.
I taste the sweetness of your name,
A love that's burning, never tame.

I wonder how you'll laugh or cry,
Will you reach for stars in the sky?
I hear you in the quiet night,
A love so pure, a guiding light.

I feel you in the air I breathe,
In every thought, in every need.
A love unseen, yet here it stays—
A bond that lasts through all our days.

CHAPTER FOUR

"The Waiting Game"

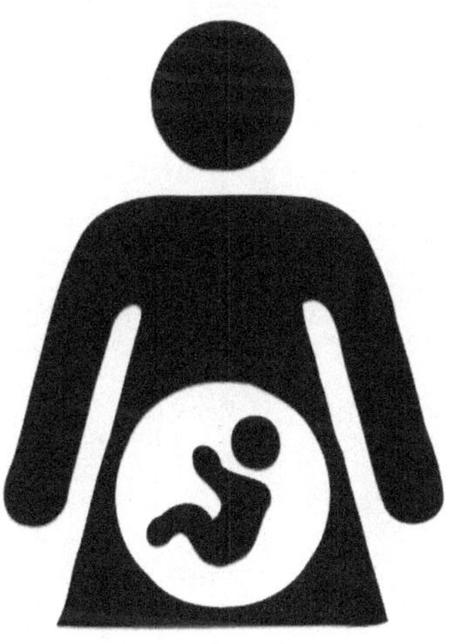

Counting the Days

Each day drags, yet flies so fast,
A rhythm steady, yet outclassed.
I count the days, the hours too,
A growing hope, a love so true.

I feel the wait, it pulls, it bends,
The days, the nights, no clear end.
The taste of time is bittersweet,
A dance of longing, hearts that beat.

I hear your movement, soft and shy,
A secret song that floats nearby.
I see your world, a distant gleam,
But soon, my love, you'll be my dream.

Nursery Dreams

The crib stands still, a place to grow,
A tiny space for you to know.
I taste the wood, the paint, the air,
A dream of you is everywhere.

The room is ready, soft and bright,
A world of warmth, a future light.
I feel the flutter deep inside,
As you prepare for this first ride.

I see your world with open eyes,
A place where love and hope arise.
The nursery hums a quiet tune,
For you to come, and find your room.

The Mix of Ready

I'm ready now, or so I think,
To welcome you, my heart does sink.
The days grow long, yet seem so sweet,
I'm nervous, yet I feel complete.

I taste the fear, I taste the joy,
A love that's pure, yet unknown toy.
I hear the ticking of the clock,
A sound so soft, it makes me rock.

I feel the flutter deep inside,
A promise kept, a love untried.
I see your face in every thought,
In every dream, in every lot.

The Pause Before

The world is still, the air is thick,
A pause between the clock's quick tick.
I feel the wait, it holds me tight,
The rush of day, the quiet night.

I taste the silence in the room,
A quiet hum, a growing bloom.
I hear your breath, soft as air,
A silent prayer, a whispered prayer.

I see the future, unclear, unknown,
Yet in my heart, your love has grown.
The pause before, the final wait,
I welcome you—my love, my fate.

A Thousand Wonders

A thousand wonders fill my mind,
What will you be, what will I find?
I count the days with hopeful eyes,
A mix of joy, of small goodbyes.

I taste the air, it's sweet, it's long,
The rhythm's slow, but still so strong.
I hear your whispers, soft and true,
A song of life that sings of you.

I feel your presence, soft and clear,
A love that waits, a love sincere.
The days will pass, the time will come,
And soon you'll be my morning sun.

CHAPTER FIVE

"Labor of Love"

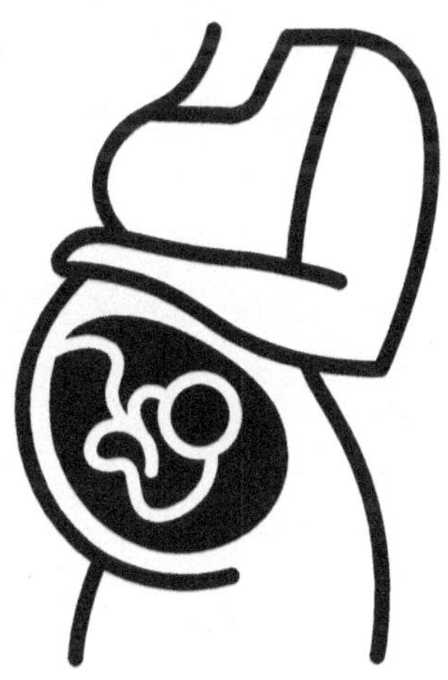

The Strength Within

The pain is sharp, the rhythm strong,
A pulse that beats, a heartbeat's song.
I taste the air, it feels so thick,
Each breath a push, each moment quick.

The waves are high, they crash and swell,
I feel the fire, I feel the hell.
But deep within, a strength I find,
A love so pure, a heart aligned.

I hear your cry, so clear, so near,
A voice that wipes away the fear.
In your first breath, the world is new,
A labor's end, but love's breakthrough.

The Final Push

The room is quiet, save for me,
A race against what's yet to be.
I feel the weight, the pull, the strain,
A force of nature in my brain.

I taste the fear, the sweat, the grit,
A moment where the stars must fit.
I hear the words, the cries, the call,
Each breath a step, each pain a wall.

But then, oh then, you enter through,
A life that's formed, a love that's true.
Your first cry rings, a song divine,
The world is yours, the world is mine.

In the Quiet Before

The silence lingers, thick with heat,
The air so close, the world on repeat.
I taste the sweat, a bitter taste,
But still, my body holds its grace.

I feel the strength, the tension rise,
A power vast as endless skies.
The pain, the push, the steady pace,
Each breath a prayer, a holy space.

And then the cry, so loud, so clear,
The joy, the love, the end is near.
I see you now, a life so bright,
A labor of love, my heart alight.

The Triumph of You

With every breath, I find my might,
A strength that burns, a steady fight.
I taste the salt, I feel the burn,
But through the pain, I start to learn.

I hear the words, the gentle cheer,
I feel the world, I see you near.
The strength within, it lifts me high,
As I prepare for you to fly.

Then in a moment, loud and clear,
Your cry bursts forth, a sound so dear.
And in that cry, the world stands still,
A love that time cannot distill.

The First Cry

The pain is sharp, yet strangely sweet,
Each moment builds, each pulse a beat.
I taste the heat of sweat and tears,
A battle fought throughout the years.

I hear your cry, a song so pure,
The pain recedes, the heart feels sure.
I see your face, so small, so bright,
A treasure held in gentle light.

I feel the joy, the love, the grace,
A world reborn in your embrace.
The labor ends, but love begins,
A new life born, a world within.

CHAPTER SIX

"First Breath, First Cry"

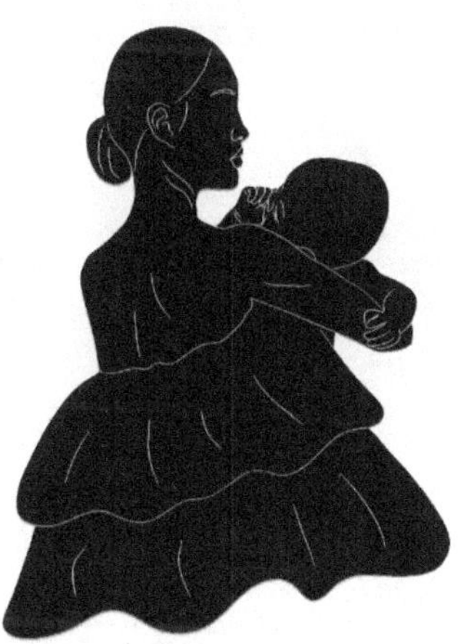

The First Touch

I hold you close, my arms embrace,
Your tiny hands, your perfect face.
I taste the air, so soft, so sweet,
A bond is formed with every beat.

I feel your warmth, your tiny skin,
A new life starts, a love begins.
I hear your cry, a sound so true,
A melody that's just for you.

I see the world in your bright eyes,
A love that never tells goodbyes.
In this first touch, I find my soul,
With you, my love, I am made whole.

The Power of Your Cry

The room is still, then fills with sound,
A cry that echoes all around.
I taste the salt, the tears I've shed,
As joy and awe fill my head.

I feel the pulse, the rush, the wave,
A moment fierce, so raw, so brave.
I hear your voice, a call so pure,
A power strong, so vast, so sure.

I see your face, a miracle here,
A love that rises, free of fear.
With your first cry, the world reborn,
A mother's love, from night to dawn.

First Breath, First Love

I hold you close, my heart does race,
A life so small, yet full of grace.
I taste the joy, so sweet, so deep,
A love that wakes from peaceful sleep.

I feel the magic in the air,
A love so deep, beyond compare.
I hear the world, a soft embrace,
As you begin your first sweet grace.

I see the future in your eyes,
A bond that never, ever dies.
With your first breath, I start to see,
The mother's love, eternally.

A Mother's Tears

Your first breath fills the air with light,
A tear slips down, pure and bright.
I taste the salt of joy and fear,
A love that brings a silent tear.

I feel your warmth against my chest,
My heart swells large, my soul feels blessed.
I hear the world stop, and in that pause,

I see you breathe, my heart in awe.
A tear falls soft, but full of grace,
For in your eyes, I see my place.
With you, my love, I'll always be,
The mother of eternity.

The First Miracle

Your tiny hand, your fragile frame,
A life so pure, a love untamed.
I taste the joy, I taste the sweet,
As your heart and mine do meet.

I feel the wonder, soft and true,
The first of many moments new.
I hear your cry, a song, a sound,
A miracle that's truly found.

I see you there, so full of light,
The world grows bright, my heart takes flight.
In your first breath, in your first cry,
A mother's love will never die.

CHAPTER SEVEN

"Tiny Hands, Endless Love"

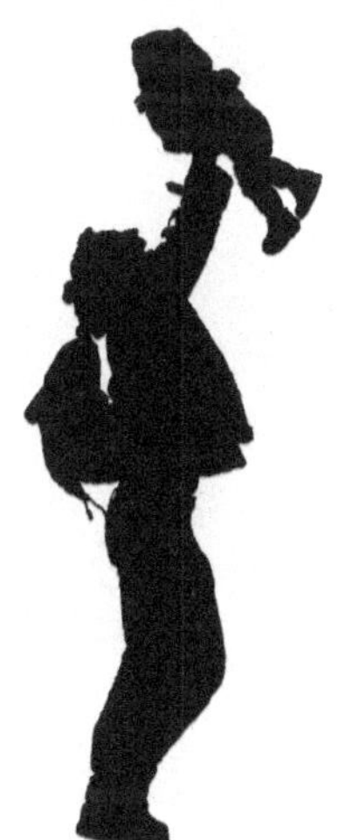

Tiny Hands, Big Heart

I gaze at your hands, so small, so sweet,
Tiny fingers, so soft, so neat.
I taste the love in every breath,
A bond so deep, no room for death.

I feel your grip, so warm, so sure,
A love that's constant, kind, and pure.
I hear the silence, calm and deep,
As you rest, my heart does weep.

I see the world through your wide eyes,
A world of wonder, no goodbyes.
In your tiny hands, I find my soul,
A love that makes me feel whole.

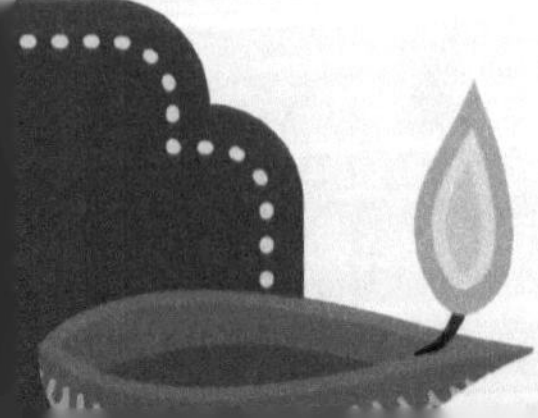

Sleepless Nights

The night is long, the world is still,
Yet here I am, with love to fill.
I taste the tired, sweet and worn,
But in your arms, I'm reborn.

I feel the weight of every cry,
Yet in your gaze, I see the sky.
I hear your soft and gentle sound,
A tiny heartbeat, love unbound.

I see the moon, the stars so bright,
But all I need is you tonight.
Though sleepless nights may leave me torn,
In your arms, I'm never worn.

A Quiet Moment

I hold you close, you rest your head,
In this moment, love is spread.
I taste the warmth of your soft skin,
A love so deep, a love within.

I feel your breath, a soft, sweet sigh,
As you drift off, I close my eyes.
I hear the world outside, it fades,
But here with you, time never wades.

I see your face, so calm, so dear,
In your peace, I have no fear.
A quiet moment, pure and sweet,
My heart is full, my soul complete.

Midnight Feeding

The moonlight shines, the room is still,
You drink your fill, I feel the thrill.
I taste the love, so soft, so near,
A bond so true, a bond so dear.

I feel the warmth, your tiny hand,
As you suckle, I understand.
I hear your hum, so soft, so light,
A melody that soothes the night.

I see the world, but all I need,
Is you and me, this perfect deed.
A midnight feeding, sweet and slow,
A love that only mothers know.

The Weight of Love

Your tiny hands, they hold my heart,
Each little grasp, a work of art.
I taste the joy, so bittersweet,
As love and life in me repeat.

I feel the weight of every cry,
But still, I hold you close, so high.
I hear your voice, your tiny plea,
A song of love, so wild and free.

I see the stars, the world's still wide,
But in your eyes, I find my guide.
With tiny hands, you hold my soul,
A love that makes me feel whole.

CHAPTER EIGHT

"Becoming Us"

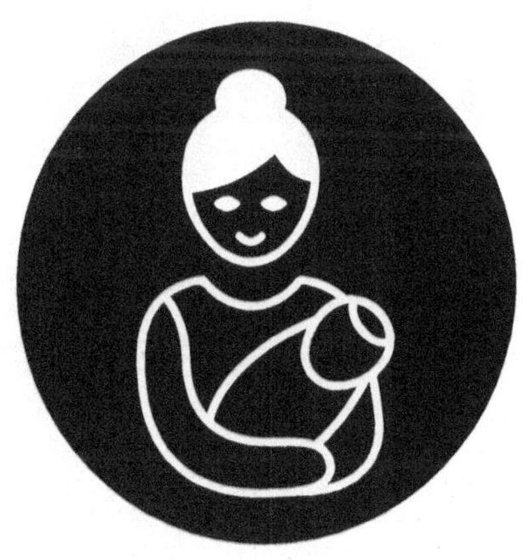

Partners in Love

In the quiet moments, we find our way,
Hand in hand, through night and day.
I taste the sweetness of shared trust,
In this journey, love is a must.

I feel your hand, so firm, so kind,
A partner's heart, intertwined.
I hear your voice, calm and near,
Assurance through each lingering fear.

I see the light in your tired eyes,
In your gaze, no need for disguise.
Together, we become more than we were,
Partners in love, hearts a blur.

Learning Together

We stumble, we fall, but still, we rise,
Learning together, no compromise.
I taste the salt of tears once shed,
But in your arms, I'm always led.

I feel the shift of love's embrace,
The growing pains of a slower pace.
I hear the lessons we both teach,
In every word, in every reach.

I see us change, as time goes by,
Stronger than we ever thought we'd fly.
Learning together, hand in hand,
Through every challenge, we still stand.

A New Rhythm

The world spins round, a dance so sweet,
A new rhythm, with each heartbeat.
I taste the sweetness of your kiss,
In moments of chaos, we find bliss.

I feel the change, the quiet beat,
Of our new rhythm, steady, neat.
I hear the laughter, soft and clear,
As we find our way through every fear.

I see the sunrise, a new day born,
In this new life, we are reborn.
Finding our rhythm, one step at a time,
In love's sweet melody, we climb.

Strength in Vulnerability

We are fragile, yet so strong,
In vulnerability, we belong.
I taste the sting of tears once shed,
But in our hearts, love is fed.

I feel the weight, the joy, the pain,
In every loss, in every gain.
I hear your heart beat next to mine,
A song of love, perfectly aligned.

I see us grow, with each new test,
Through vulnerability, we find rest.
In our weakness, we find strength anew,
Together, love, me and you.

Becoming Us

The world shifts, but we remain,
In love, we weather joy and pain.
I taste the hope in every breath,
In this partnership, no fear, no death.

I feel your warmth, your guiding hand,
Together we walk, through shifting sand.
I hear the echoes of our song,
A love so deep, so fierce, so strong.

I see the future, bright and clear,
With you beside me, I have no fear.
Becoming us, with every day,
A love that's here, and will always stay.

CHAPTER NINE

"The Mother Within"

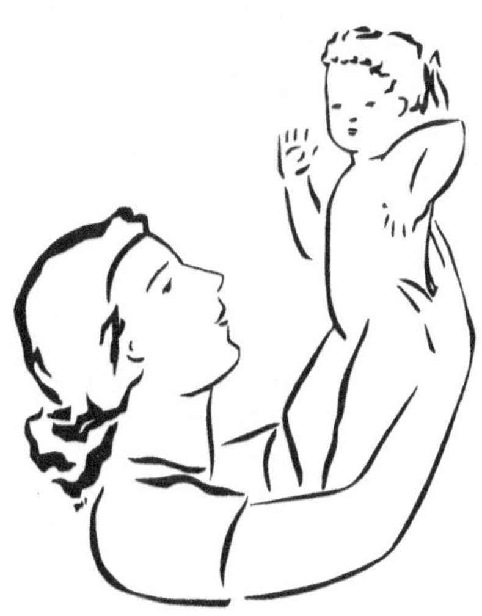

The Loss and the Gain

In the quiet dawn, I softly see,
The mother I am, the me I used to be.
I taste the salt of dreams once bright,
Now faded, lost, like the starless night.

I feel the pull of who I was,
And who I've become, without a cause.
I hear my heart, both old and new,
A blend of love and grief, it's true.

I see the strength, a fire inside,
A woman reborn, with nothing to hide.
The mother within, so fierce and free,
A mix of joy and loss, but complete in me.

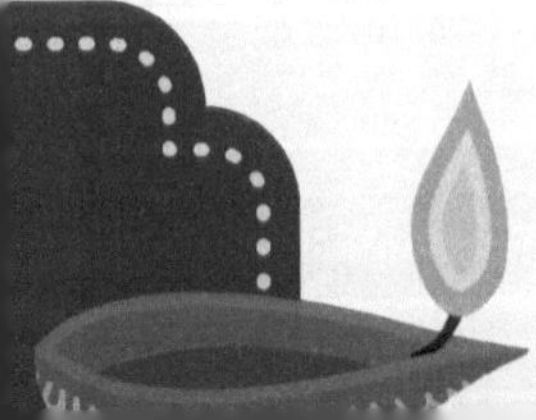

Strength in Silence

I taste the bitterness of forgotten dreams,
But in my chest, the heart still screams.
The mother within, so strong and wild,
A resilience born with every child.

I feel the weight of love's embrace,
The endless care, the constant grace.
I hear the whispers of my soul,
Calling me back to make me whole.

I see the power of my hands,
Strong enough to help them stand.
In silence, strength takes root and grows,
The mother within, with love that glows.

Becoming More

Once I was only me, so free,
Now I'm more than I used to be.
I taste the change, a sweetness deep,
As dreams evolve from those I keep.

I feel the joy, the growing pains,
In motherhood's steady, sweet reigns.
I hear my voice, both calm and bold,
Telling stories, both new and old.

I see the woman, strong and new,
With hands to heal, a heart so true.
Becoming more, I embrace it all,
Motherhood's rise, with each new call.

Resilient Roots

I taste the earth, the roots that bind,
A mother's strength in every find.
The mother within, so fierce and true,
Resilient as the morning dew.

I feel the love, the boundless fire,
A passion that will never tire.
I hear the rhythm of my soul,
A heartbeat steady, strong, and whole.

I see the future, wide and free,
A life reborn, a destiny.
With roots so deep, so strong, so clear,
The mother within, forever near.

Embracing Change

I taste the sweetness of what's new,
In every step, in every view.
The mother within, a force to see,
A new identity, wild and free.

I feel the pull of who I was,
But embrace the now without a pause.
I hear the echoes of the past,
But I am here, and I will last.

I see the woman I've become,
A mother, strong, a beating drum.
Embracing change, I rise, I grow,
A force of love, forever aglow.

CHAPTER TEN

"Eternal Love"

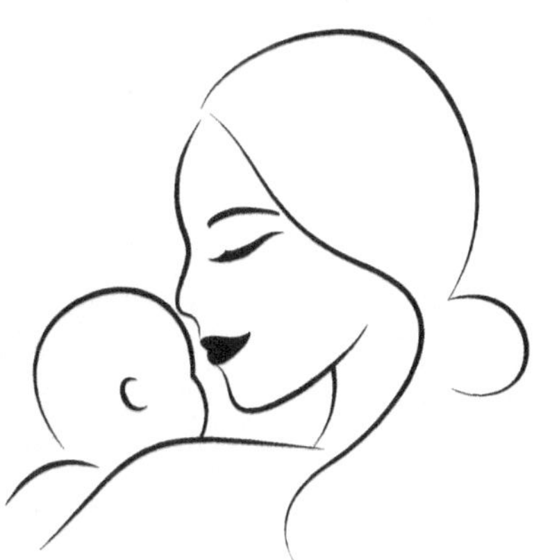

The First Steps Recalled

I taste the tears of joy that fell,
As I watched you grow, I could tell,
From first breath to your first cry,
You became my reason to fly.

I feel the weight of every day,
Each moment precious, each step, a way.
From sleepless nights to sunny skies,
A journey built of love's ties.

I hear your laughter, sweet and clear,
A melody that draws me near.
Looking back, I see it all,
Your first steps, and my heart's call.

A Love Letter to You

My darling child, my gift so pure,
In your embrace, my heart is sure.
I taste your sweetness, soft and bright,
A love that shines, a guiding light.

I feel the warmth of every touch,
The softest hands that mean so much.
I hear your voice, both calm and wild,
You'll always be my precious child.

I see the future, wide and free,
All that you will one day be.
This bond, eternal, we will share,
A love that's constant, always there.

Gratitude's Embrace

I taste the quiet in the night,
Grateful for your love so bright.
I feel the magic in each sigh,
A mother's joy, reaching high.

I hear the whispers in the breeze,
That tell me you will always be,
A part of me, through every storm,
A love that's timeless, pure, and warm.

I see the future in your eyes,
The hope that never fades or dies.
Thank you, my love, for all you are,
You're my guiding light, my shining star.

Forever Ours

I taste the sweetness of our past,

A love that's built, forever to last.

I feel the rhythm of your soul,

In every heartbeat, you make me whole.

I hear your dreams in whispered songs,

A melody that carries on.

You're the echo of my heart,

The beginning of a brand-new start.

I see the promise in your gaze,

A future filled with love and grace.

Forever ours, this bond so true,

A mother's love, eternal and new.

To the Future, With Love

I taste the salt of days long gone,
The moments fleeting, but we carry on.
I feel the love that time can't take,
A bond that only grows, never to break.

I hear the future calling near,
With hope and joy, we have no fear.
You are my heart, my dream, my song,
With you, my love will always belong.

I see you growing, wide and free,
The world at your feet, the sky, the sea.
My eternal love, my guiding light,
I'll stand by you, day and night.

Final Note

Dear Reader,

Thank you for choosing Becoming Mother and allowing my words to accompany you on this profound journey into motherhood. It means so much to know these poems have been a part of your experience.

If this collection resonated with you or brought comfort, I'd love to hear your thoughts. Your reflections not only brighten my day but also help other readers discover this book.

Please consider leaving a review on the platform where you found it—it makes a meaningful difference. Thank you for your support and for sharing this journey with me.

With gratitude,
Taylor Quill

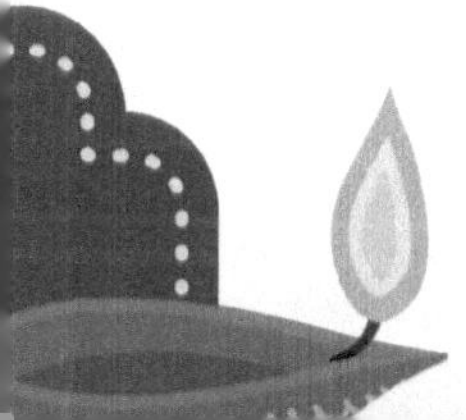

About the Author

Taylor Quill is a contemporary poet and writer known for her evocative and heartfelt explorations of love, resilience, and personal growth. Born and raised in the Pacific Northwest, Taylor draws inspiration from the natural world and the complexities of human experience.

With a background in creative writing and psychology, Taylor's work is infused with empathy, vulnerability, and a deep understanding of the human condition. Her poetry invites readers to reflect on their own journeys, embracing the beauty and complexity of life.

Dare to Love Again, Taylor's debut poetry collection, is a testament to her own experiences with heartbreak, healing, and the transformative power of love. When not writing, Taylor enjoys hiking, journaling, and sipping coffee in quiet cafes.

www.ingramcontent.com/pod-product-compliance
Lightning Source LLC
Chambersburg PA
CBHW051820130726

47987CB00003B/1347